THE
EPILEPTIC WARRIOR PRINCESS
- LIFE WITH EPILEPSY

HOW TO MANAGE, UNDERSTAND AND
OVERCOME STRUGGLES THAT
COME WITH IT ON A REGULAR BASIS

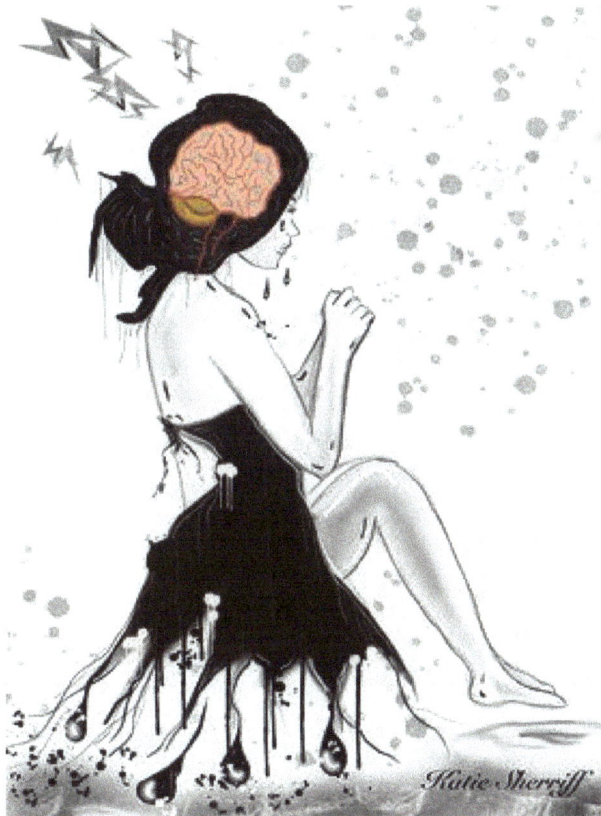

Katie Sherriff

By

TAMARA AND CHESS SIMEUNOVIC

Dedication

To my mum Sanja Simeunovic, Dada, Chess, London Book Publishing, Professor Ley Sander, Dr Anne Anderson, Katie Sheriff, Carolyn, Dom, Grace, Mandy and Lucy, and all the readers.

Thank you so much for helping me with my book journey. Without your help and support throughout life, this book would not have been possible. Thank you so much for making my dream of raising understanding and awareness of life with epilepsy come to life. Thank you for supporting me with my condition, for publishing this book and choosing to read it. This journey would not have been possible without you.

Acknowledgement

I wish to thank my mum for bringing me up, supporting me throughout life and risking her own life to bring me up, taking care of me and supporting me throughout most aspects all my life despite it not being easy most of the time. I wish to thank my stunning non-blood sisters Carolyn, Mandy, Lucy and Grace and my non-blood brother Dom especially Dom and Carolyn and Grace for supporting me through dark times, believing in me and understanding me when no one else did. Carolyn and Dom along with Grace helped me not only throughout the years emotionally with bullying and with my relationships, but have been the closest family and most loyal, loving, understanding, empathic and supportive friends and siblings I could ask for and helped me out of the darkness when I felt hopeless, like I was a lost cause, defeated and depressed. They helped me through thick and thin see the light at the end of the tunnel as well as helped me learn new talents in writing books and learning to draw and be creative as well as learning to sing and explore new talents and discover new areas of life I was too afraid to explore before, along with learning IT skills. At times when I felt I had no one, and had lost the most precious people in my life, they were my rock and my support. Mandy and Lucy have been so supportive and helped me also realize there is light at end of the tunnel and to keep up my strength and keep battling on. My lovely GP Dr Anne Anderson and my neurologist Professor Ley Sander have been the most supportive and greatest medical professionals despite me being a complicated patient with difficult epilepsy and never once gave up on me. They taught me to never give up on dreams and future despite my condition and that nothing is out of reach as long as I believe in myself which is why I always aimed high in life and kept fighting. Thank you to Katie Sherriff for doing the illustrations in this book-your talent is amazing and I am proud for you to have done this journey of creating this book with me. I also wish to thank London Book Publishing for making this book come to life and for believing in me as a first-time author- without you-this book would not have been published and brought to life. I acknowledge everyone who reads this book and thank you for recognizing it and the importance of raising awareness of epilepsy and the difficulties faced having the condition with this book. Thank you so much Lots of love Tamara and Chess Simeunovic

Table of Contents

Introduction

Welcome to my book about living with epilepsy

I have had epilepsy since I was 2 years old and have had several types and undergone various different medications over the years including some with bad side effects. Sadly, as I lived my life with epilepsy, I realized how much misunderstanding about the condition there is from all aspects of society from the ones closest to you, to doctors to employers etc. I got fed up of the stigma and of epilepsy not being understood well as a neurological condition particularly when it can be life threatening and how people that have it are overlooked or mistreated or misunderstood by others in society because of their lack of understanding of the condition and the psychological and behavioural aspects and struggles that come with it. Epilepsy does not just affect the people with the condition but also those close to the sufferer and as they sadly do not teach it in schools and as research on medications is constantly developing, I thought to write this book to help people with condition, parents, partners, medical staff, employers, friends and family, and society in general understand the condition better and learn how to manage it so that the sufferer is not misunderstood or mistreated by others in society just because of pure ignorance and lack of knowledge about the condition. It will also hopefully help sufferers realize they are not alone and learn how to adapt to certain situations in society so they can manage their condition better and hopefully be seizure free like me one day. I hope this book helps everyone and I hope knowledge of the condition improves so sufferers don't have to struggle so much in life. A lot of people take for granted a lot of the things epileptics cannot do alone and I want to make society realize how hard life is with this neurological condition and for society to never take anything in life for granted because epilepsy can occur at any point in life to anybody and it is very hard to cure and live with

Various Types of Epilepsy, Symptoms/ What They Look Like and Areas of Brain Affected

There are many different types of epilepsy and therefore different types of seizures. This depends on which area or areas of the brain is affected. If only one lobe/area of the brain is affected, then the seizures will be much less aggressive and there is less chance of injury to the individual. It will also mean the individual will likely take lower dosages of medication required and be less restricted to the things that they can do in everyday life than those with more severe types of epilepsy and seizures. In this chapter, I will attempt to explain the most common types of epilepsy and seizures, the areas of the brain affected and the symptoms/what seizures look like in each type as well as how each type affects the individual. I hope this helps not only carers and parents, but especially those who have little to no knowledge of epilepsy and seizures and no understanding of the condition to understand and realize what the individual is going through and how to help them instead of misjudging them. This I feel is especially important for HR and other employment based individuals as well as friends of the individual.

Simple Partial Focal Seizures

Simple partial seizures usually occur only in one area of the brain-the temporal lobe. The temporal lobe is the area of the brain responsible for processing sensory input, long-term memory, emotion association, visual memory, and language comprehension. Because only the temporal lobe is affected, and no other lobes are usually affected in these type of seizures, there is less damage in the brain and the individual usually remains conscious whilst having a simple partial focal seizure.

People with simple partial focal seizures will get auras. They will not lose consciousness. These auras can be brief headaches, feeling like its groundhog day where events seem to repeat themselves, heightened senses or unusual tastes or smells, brief stiffness or brief twitching.

Complex Focal Seizures

These can occur either in the frontal lobe or the temporal lobe. Complex focal seizures that occur in the frontal lobe of the brain tend to last shorter than those that occur in the temporal lobe. If complex focal seizures occur in both frontal and temporal lobes, these develop into generalized seizures which are more dangerous and more aggressive than focal and partial seizures occurring in only one lobe of the brain. The seizures last for about 30 seconds and 3 minutes but because these seizures occur mostly in the temporal lobe, memory loss and sensory information is affected and the individual will be tired and confused for a few hours afterwards. Until they recover their memory and come out of confusion, they are unlikely to remember names of their medication when asked by paramedics so will need help in this area. Complex partial and focal seizures tend to occur more regularly in individuals who have had a previous head injury, stroke, tumour or brain infection.

During a complex partial seizure, individuals lose sense of awareness and make random body movements, such as:

- lipsmacking
- handrubbing
- making random noises/loud cries
- moving your arms around randomly and uncontrollably
- picking at clothes or fiddling with objects without being aware of doing so

They will not be able to respond to anyone else during the seizure due to lack of awareness and being spaced out and they will not have any memory of the seizure and what they were doing.

Tonic Clonic Seizures

This type of seizure is a generalized seizure type and therefore occurs in both areas of the brain and therefore in more than one lobe and imbalances in the neurotransmitter activity to the brain

This is the second most dangerous type of epilepsy after staticus epilepticus due to the violent shaking and injuries caused as well as the length of the seizure where the brain is being depleted of oxygen during the seizure and if the seizure lasts too long, it can sometimes cause brain damage. The individual will lose consciousness and body goes stiff and they will fall to the floor-the tonic phase. Then the body enters the clonic phase immediately after this where the body starts to jerk, shake violently and the individual will be unaware of what is happening. They may lose control of their bladder, severely injure themselves and have concussion or head injury. It is important to remove all potentially harmful objects such as tables, anything glass made, any knives/sharp objects out of the way, ideally before the seizure if possible. If this cannot be done, do it during the seizure to prevent further injury before calling paramedics and putting individual in recovery position to regain breathing and consciousness when they come around from the seizure. Individuals will have memory loss, be concussed, have severe headaches and need to rest and recover post seizure and may need hospital treatment for injuries to head, face, spine (depending how they have fallen and what injuries were sustained). It is ideal to have a carer or someone individual trusts beside them and to supervise them to help doctors understand what happened and to help individual recollect what happened

Myoclonic Seizures

Myoclonic-means muscle jerking. In these seizures, the individual's muscles jerk and shake violently and uncontrollably usually arms and legs (although I have my head shaking too) until seizure stops.

Individuals can be conscious or unconscious (in my case unconscious) and seizure can be brief of 2mins but mine have known to be 5mins or longer. Dangerous objects should be moved away, paramedics called if seizure lasts longer than 3mins. Individuals may sustain injury to head, face, neck and body due to the fall and may have memory loss and concussion. They usually need to rest the rest of the day to recover their brain and body from seizure and will take few days for muscles and body to recover from injuries.

Absences/Petite Mal	With absences/petite mal seizures, the epileptic looks like they are daydreaming or in a trance/staring into space very briefly. During this time, they cannot hear what you are saying to them but are still conscious. They usually last a few seconds and are the shortest lasting of all seizures.
Tonic Seizures	The muscles become stiff as though numb/paralyzed briefly. Often epileptics with tonic seizures lose their balance, fall over and cause injury to themselves due to brief numbness/paralysis in their muscles and inability to control their muscles and joints.

Clonic Seizures	Epileptics with clonic type seizures will jerk and shake but will not go stiff in their muscles unlike the tonic seizures. It is common to lose consciousness, be confused and sometimes have injury. The seizures will last a few minutes before regaining consciousness. Injury to tongue, head and confusion and brief concussion is common.
Atonic Seizures	Atonic seizures cause all your muscles to suddenly relax, so you may fall to the ground. They tend to be very brief (about 2mins) and you'll usually be able to get up again straight away although you may be a bit confused for a brief while post seizure.

Status Epilepticus	Status epilepticus is the name for any seizure that lasts a long time (longer than 8mins), or a series of seizures where the person does not regain consciousness in between. It is the most dangerous type of seizures and epilepsy to have, as the person can die from this type of seizure due to amount of damage caused in the brain and how long the seizures occur for due to depletion of oxygen and blood from the brain with each passing minute the seizure lasts for. If you see a person having a status epilepticus seizure, it is vital to call 999 immediately due to the harm the seizure poses to the individual

Various Anti-Epileptic Medications I Have Been Prescribed and Side Effects Including Some Unusual Side Effects Not Always Listed and Told About

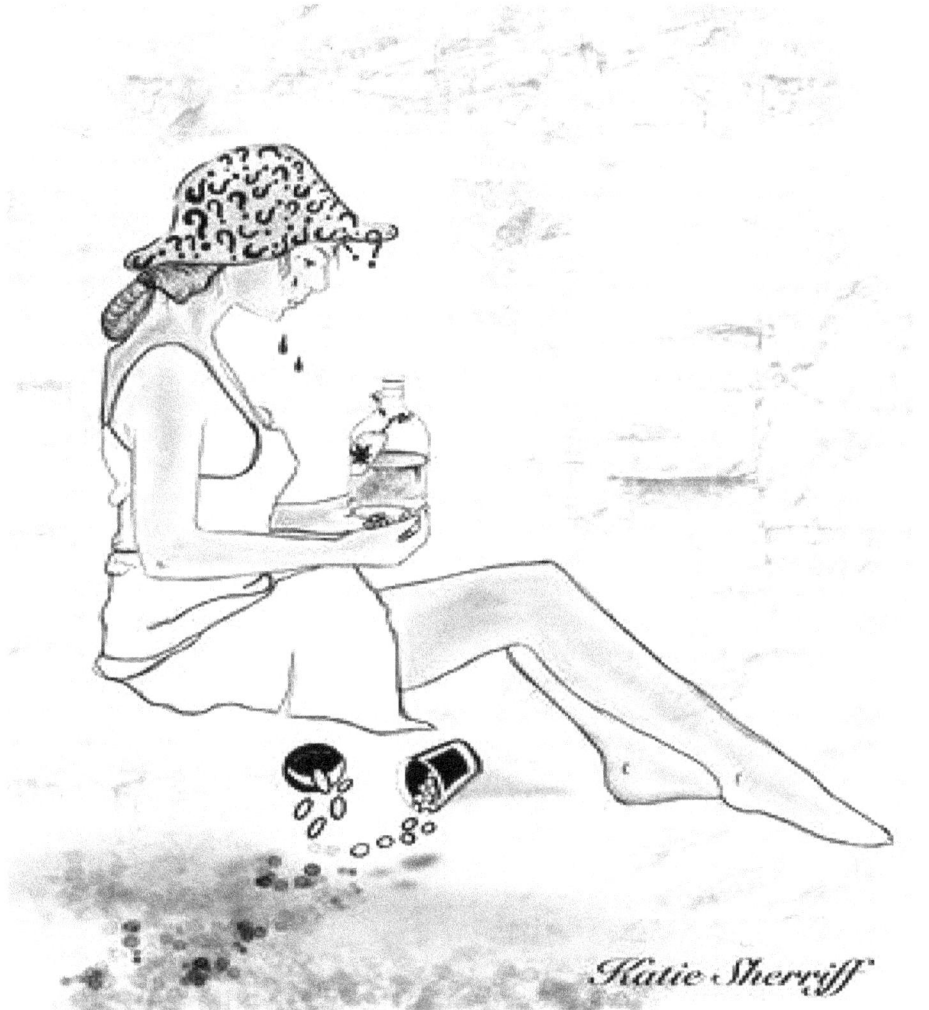

Katie Sherriff

THE EPILEPTIC WARRIOR PRINCESS

SCIENTIFIC NAME OF MEDICATION	COMMON NAME FOR MEDICATION	SIDE EFFECTS LISTED FOR THE MEDICATION	UNUSUAL SIDE EFFECTS I EXPERIENCED
CANNABIS OIL	CBD OIL		OVERFERTILE, WEIGHTLOSS, FATIGUE,
BRIVIACETAM	BRIVIACT	DROWZINESS SEDATION DIZZINESS FATIGUE NAUSEA VOMITING LOSS OF BALANCE LOSSOF COORDINATION CONSTIPATION IRRITABILITY	ANXIETY, DEPRESSION, HEIGHTENED SENSES, PHOTOSENSITIVITY
FYCOMPA	PERAMPANEL	WEIGHT GAIN VERTIGO ANXIETY ABDOMINAL PAIN	COMMUNICATION PROBLEMS VOMITING CONSTANTLY,

		BRUISING HEADACHE MUSCLE COORDINATION PROBLEMS DIZZINESS SLEEPINESS NAUSEA/ VOMITING IRRITABILITY	HEIGHTENED SENSES
ZONEGRAN	ZONISAMIDE	LIGHT-HEADEDNESS LOSS OF APPETITE DOUBLE VISION DIARRHEA INSOMNIA DIZZINESS DROWZINESS WEIGHTLOSS	ANOREXIA HEIGHTENED SENSES
LEVETIRACETAM	KEPPRA	DIZZINESS AGGRESSION ANXIETY IRRATIBILITY NERVOUSNESS SEETHING RAGE	MOODSWINGS, BAD TEMPER, EAD, PERSONALITY DISORDER

		UNCONTROLLED ANGER SUICIDAL TENDENCIES DEPRESSION LOSS OF APPETITE	
ZARONTIN	ETHOSUXIMIDE	CRAMPS HICCUPS INCREASED HAIR GROWTH VOMITING NAUSEA DISCOMFORT IN CHEST, THROAT AND UPPER STOMACH SLUGGISHNESS TIREDNESS	CRAMPS HAIR LOSS LOSS OF APPETITE TIREDNESS
EPILIM	SODIUM VALPROATE	BLEEDING TENDER GUMS ABDOMINAL PAIN/CRAMPS WEIGHT GAIN PROLONGED PERIODS HEADACHE	UNABLE TO GAIN WEIGHT, OVERFERTILE, MEMORY ISSUES, LONGER TO HEAL FROM INJURIES, HEAVY BRUISING

		CHANGES IN APPETITE DIARRHOEA VOMITING BONE WEAKNESS	

Diet and Epilepsy

People with epilepsy usually are a bit sensitive to certain foods as a result of the medication they are taking. This is the main reason why epileptics should not drink alcohol, too much sugar impacts the electrical state in the neurons in the brain and can cause migraine like headaches which can worsen frequency of seizures. High salt intake is also bad for epileptics as it causes increased heartrate, which sends extra electric impulses throughout the body and to the brain which can make seizures worse. This is why processed foods and high salt foods are not ideal for people with epilepsy.

Some people with epilepsy are told to follow the Atkins diet but I found this extremely restrictive and stodgy as you are not allowed any carbohydrates whatsoever and I could not do without pasta or rice at least once a week. Also the Atkins diet puts you at risk of high cholesterol levels which can put you at risk of strokes if fat globules form in your brain. This is why I follow the ketogenic diet which helps me keep weight off as I get older, and although it is restrictive in some areas such as no fried foods are allowed, no processed sugar, certain carbohydrates are allowed so I am happy to have quinoa and lamb with avocado and tomatoes for example. I have invented some of my own keto-friendly recipes which are delicious for everyone including my lemon and coconut flavoured salmon.

Oily fish and good fats and protein rich foods are highly recommended for people with epilepsy as is not drinking too much caffeine-so energy drinks are a major no-no for epileptics as is drinking too many cups of English breakfast tea. Herbal tea is good for the brain and body and therefore encouraged-I especially have chamomile and valerian root tea at night to help me sleep as I sometimes struggle with insomnia. I also grow my own herbs in my garden for cooking and making tea including basil, jasmine, oregano, lemon verbena, chocolate mint, pineapple mint, morrocan mint, common mint, parsley, coriander, sage, rosemary, French lavender, normal lavender, lemon thyme, normal thyme and valerian root.

Epilepsy and My Young Childhood-Early and Primary School Years

I was diagnosed with petit mal epilepsy (absences) when I was two years old. After having a vaccine, I had a couple of days of high temperature. I then started staring for some seconds when playing. When talking I would just stop and then continue the sentence. I was put on sodium valproate and absences stopped. My EEG was also fine. At the age of 3 I had high temperature again and absences returned even on medication. Different medicines were tried, ethosuximide and phenobarbiturates which were very overpowering. My mum says that I was very slow and very tired.

This continued to the age of 5 when we got to England as war refugees. I was referred to a consultant in Royal Free Hospital who reduced my medication and I "woke up" but absences continued. Different medication was tried including Tegretol and I had to re-learn to walk as well as learn to speak, read and write English from scratch. Absences increased but despite this I was doing very well at school. My work was very good even though English was my second language which I had to learn from scratch when I got to the UK and I was praised my teachers for my excellent spelling, grammar, punctuation, reading, writing and speaking skills.

Bullying started at year 2 when it was obvious that I was different than the other girls. Girls would group together to bully me. However, it got severely worse in Year 4 when I was bullied by the popular girls and in after school clubs. I felt I did not fit in and felt very lonely but also felt I could not talk to the teacher as I was terrified. It is a lot harder when you are very young and you cannot know what exact problem with your health is so you find it hard to talk about it to others, but it becomes even harder when you feel scared of someone or feel you cannot rely on people. Support in schools with health issues is vital and whilst this has improved thanks to medical research and knowledge over time with neurological health conditions, it was not there unfortunately when I attended school and so I felt I had to deal with issues alone. Nowadays, support is better, but I feel more training needs to be done with staff, employers at schools so that there is more specialized understanding of the various types of epilepsy so that teachers do not assume that "you are not paying attention". I was always a quiet, hardworking person who never liked being popular. I had to do nativity play and play the pear tree in "12 days of Christmas" despite not feeling comfortable with performing due to my shy nature. My teachers were lovely in infants school and I met one of my best friends Carolyn who I see as a sister and her husband is like a brother to me now. We helped each other out at school through social challenges and helped me cope through school a lot as well as helped me emotionally and with my health as my epilepsy was not as bad thanks to the calming influence of my friend which decreased my stress levels. My mum helped me as much as she could but I did a lot of the work myself. I had to learn to rely on myself from a young age.

At that time, my Mum decided to ask for the second opinion and I was referred to Great Ormond Street Hospital. I was their patient until the age of 16. Professor Neville, my consultant, also noticed that my fine motor skills were not as they should have been and diagnosed me with developmental dyspraxia. It took years of exercise and patience to improve my writing and motor skills but with help of my Mum I did it. My motor skills were never good with sports but I was fine with musical instruments which I loved, attended Harrow Young Musicians and enjoyed reading, being in garden, having pets, baking and cooking, and digging fossils out of clay before making dinosaurs out of them.

Secondary School, College and University Years

Education can be tough and stressful for most teenagers but especially those with special needs or disabilities despite it being rewarding at the end. You have to deal with personal problems such as changes within yourself e.g. puberty and hormonal changes- which can make epilepsy worse, deal with bullying and attempting to socialize and make friends, but if you are introverted and awkward, this makes it even more challenging. Alongside this, there are challenges with trying to achieve best possible grades in all subjects even when you struggle with certain subjects and the stress of homework and exams. If you have autism or ADHD or other mental health condition alongside your epilepsy, it is a major challenge and stressful being forced to wear uniform you do not feel comfortable in, dealing with puberty, trying to make friends, dealing with bullying whilst trying to keep your health good and trying to keep stress low in order to achieve best grades you can.

During secondary school, I had only a few friends and was quite shy and awkward, but I had good concentration in classes and worked hard all the time as well as doing my homework on time and achieved merits in my diary as well as got good reports from teachers all the time. I also helped the school with serving drinks at parents evening. The teachers loved me as a student and always said I was a pleasure to teach with only one saying "I will never be a good rugby player". As I was a bit like Hermione at school, I got bullied quite a lot, but the bullies were always in groups, putting daddy long legs in my shirt, throwing rubbers at me and stealing my books and bag. I lost my temper as everyone has a breaking point after a lot of bullying by same people and pushed the lead bully into the mud in front of his mates. Others saw this but my best friend Nicky backed me up as she saw how much I was bullied and how I was upset and supported me as did the teachers. Others who bullied me were jealous of my good grades. I got good GCSE grades and did okay at A-level as I found them more stressful.

At the age of 16 I was transferred to National Hospital at Queens Square under the care of Prof Sander, who is still my consultant, after 22 years. I hope he never retires, not unless he solves the mystery called "Tamara" as I am the most complicated patient he has ever had and a real mystery.

I decided to go to college after A-Levels and do BTEC in Animal Management. I really enjoyed the course and I met and made some great friends who I am still friends with today. I found the course really enjoyable although I did find some aspects of it challenging. My epilepsy did not affect me too much during this course and after completing this course, I started volunteering at Farmyard Funworld and started working at Medivet. I kept in touch with the lovely friends I made at college including Sarah, Cheryl, Louise and Hayley although sadly I lost touch completely with Hayley later, despite her visiting me in hospital. Due to stress at being dismissed from Medivet unfairly, I had to have a heart operation in 2007 which after putting defibrillator in me, my epilepsy turned from absences to grand mal seizures and I also had an anaphylactic reaction to the codeine I was given. Since then I have had grandmal seizures at least a few times a month and undergone numerous dosage and medication changes. The defibrillator battery has had to be changed every few years which has not helped my seizures so I am relieved that finally it will be taken out although the leads are now engrossed into my arteries and veins and cannot be removed.

I then went to university in Teesside in Middlesbrough to do forensics. I struggled to make friends and although I made a few lovely friends in drama society and only two from my course, there were several who took advantage of me and my intelligence. I was bullied by girls who had no clue where Bosnia was in the world and called me a "savage". I was taken advantage of and had money taken from me, had my work plagiarized and had to re-do assignments I worked hard on and struggled to be accepted in group work where teachers had to force me into groups as no one wished to work with me in practicals despite me being very methodical, analytical and excellent at solving problems. I really struggled living in halls of residence with others as they were very party-like and I wanted to focus on my work and get enough sleep. However, with loud music blaring every night, I really struggled and I had a couple of bad seizures where I had a seizure in shower and there was blood. I felt the other residents in the halls did not really care except maybe 2 of the girls, and I had no choice but to attend class despite having concussion and struggling post seizure as I was aware the class would not be repeated and I did not have any true friends I could rely on in my class at the time. I got into relationships after nights out at student union in attempt to socialize but I really struggled to get my health on track despite having support from university where someone took notes for me in class when I was not feeling post seizure able to focus and write. My teachers were lovely and I really enjoyed doing two degrees at same time alongside Drama Society and meeting lovely friends, and I was so relieved to graduate in 2013. Seizures can get worse due to stress such as tight deadlines, exams and juggling all of this as well as attending classes and attempting to maintain health. In hindsight, I should have maybe only done one degree and maybe tried to do something to de-stress and relax me even though it was hard with several noisy party animals living with you. I was always friendly towards everyone and whilst several liked me and saw me for who I was, others did not appreciate me. If I was to give advice to anyone it would be "It is the quality of friends who counts not the quantity and focus on studies always and put yourself first because no one will jump rivers for you-only you can jump rivers yourself". My mother, auntie and Nicky attended my graduation with me and we had lovely day. I got an apprenticeship shortly after in radiology at James Cook University Hospital, completed it and did teacher training afterwards. I started off doing exam invigilating and supply teaching in various schools before becoming Lecturer of Science and progressed to Course Leader and Head of Science at College. I always idolized Gus Montgomery, Gary

Weeks and Helen Tidy at university out of the lecturers and hoped I could be as good as them in teaching career. It is important to work hard and not let your medical conditions define you. Do not let epilepsy overtake you and define you and make you feel hopeless. If one door/ career shuts, accept, and try another. Where there is a will there is a way and it is important to never give up as epileptics are just as intelligent and even more so than non-epileptics- we just have a harder time displaying it due to our health and usually lack of confidence.

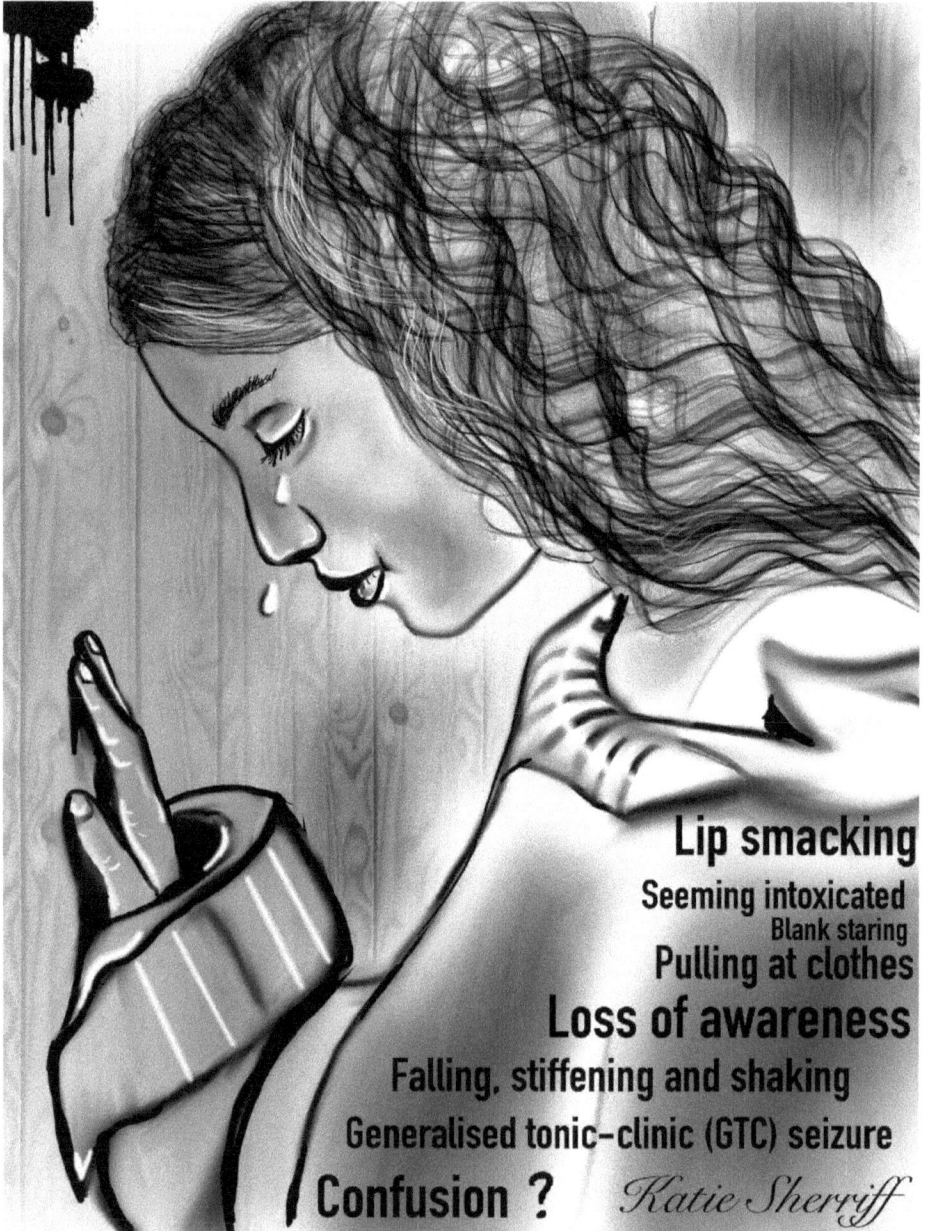

Socialization Issues with Epilepsy and How To Overcome Some of The Obstacles

A fantastic research study has been done on why and how epilepsy challenges social lives by and published on science direct which can be found in this link below for a generalized explanation

Why epilepsy challenges social life - ScienceDirect

However, here is a more personal experience of social challenges with epilepsy that I have experienced throughout life that many can relate to as well:

It is very difficult to socialize when you have epilepsy as you are misunderstood and constantly worry about having seizures in public. If you are photosensitive like myself with grandma epilepsy, then living and coping in a digital age where everything is computer reliant, cameras everywhere, sirens everywhere, and flashy strobes in theatres, cinemas, bowling alleys and practically everywhere you go is a real issue. There are no notifications before you book theatres, cinemas etc if movies, musicals etc contain flashing lights so it is always a risk as much as going to a restaurant when allergic to peanuts and hoping that none of the ingredients contain nuts nor are cooked around nuts. You have to make a difficult choice to go and risk seizure or try to protect yourself by wearing sunglasses but then being effectively blind and not able to see musical or film and relying on your hearing senses entirely instead or not attending. Every time you go out, people are so obsessed with social media and their phones, they take flashy photos everywhere and this is real issue for someone with epilepsy trying to dodge lots of phone addicts in town centres, London, at stations etc. Sirens from ambulances and police cars that go by also trigger my seizures so I have to wear sunglasses outside day and night as I never know when an ambulance or police car may pass me by. It is a constant worry and increases anxiety for those with epilepsy. This is turn makes it even harder to socialize as you are very anxious and not a social butterfly. Having to socialize and make friends is tough when complete strangers- that is what people are before you become friends- do not understand your condition and especially if you have had frequent bullying, homewrecking, and people at school did not want to hang out with you nor work with you and include you in their group. You think "what is the point"? It is very important to keep yourself safe with majority of social outings although certain, more introverted style outings such as markets, parks, museums, galleries, gardens, clubs, gyms and societies and most restaurants do not have camera/ social media addicts, strobe lighting and other seizure triggers and will have staff always to help. By going to these types of places instead will help you gain social skills by socializing with more introverted people or people who are not fans of flashy lights and help you also boost your confidence and lessen anxiety as you feel safer in these types of areas to socialize in. I recently joined Chess club as well as reading club and met like-minded individuals who do not like huge social groups but are highly intelligent and socialize better in small groups. I also attend art group that my closest friends Carolyn and Mandy arrange and do singing lessons with Grace.

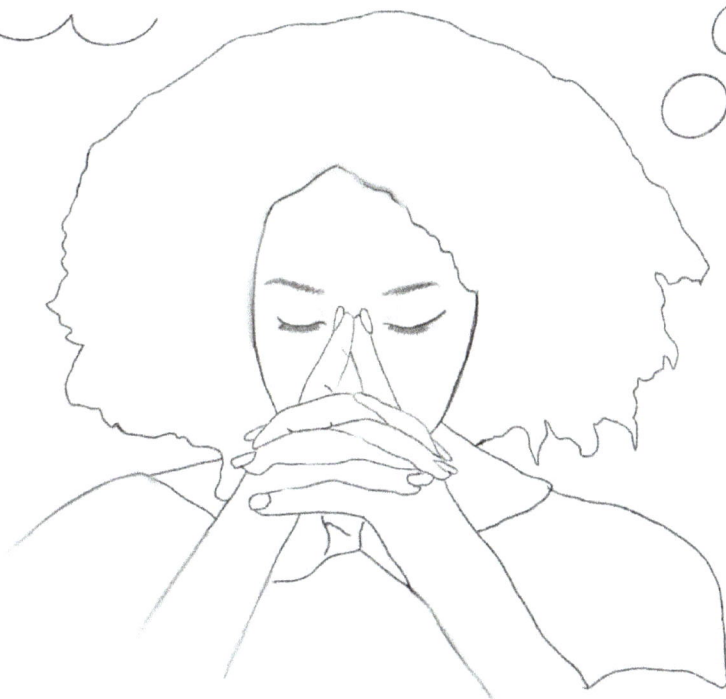

Relationship and family issues

Reduce my stress levels

Not able to get jobs

Not able to handle flashing lights

Difficulty talking about condition

Not able to take a bath or shower alone

Not being able to drive

Communication with people

Katie Sherriff

Relationship Issues

Relationships in general are hard work as they involve two individuals who are different to each other, and relationships only work if both people put equal amount of effort in. However, when you have a long-term health condition which makes you rely on your other half for certain things such as having a shower and bath in my case or driving me to places I cannot get to with my seizure alert dog or having to explain my epilepsy to strangers because of having a seizure outside in a restaurant or in a hotel or in the street, it makes things a lot harder for the both of you and can put a strain on relationships due to stress. Your partner may be unable to cope at times with certain aspects of your condition that you cannot control.

It is easy to mistake a grand mal seizure for an intoxicated individual due to people's lack of knowledge about the condition and people are quick to judge you without getting to know you. This is why I always had to be an open book and be vulnerable towards all my partners. Sadly decent guys seem to always be out of my reach and I seem to attract either narcissists, cheaters, alcoholics, drug addicts, violent people, or domestically abusive people, sex pests or man-child as these guys seem to be confident, friendly, kind, clever and intelligent, have common sense, They are approachable and the kind you wish to bring to your parents when you first meet them. They also usually have good jobs, are hardworking, usually appear to have nice friends and family and make friends easily.

However, after getting to know them better, you will find they are narcissistic and emotionally immature and that you have been living a lie whole time. You will find yourself arguing with someone who is convinced they know more about your condition than your neurologist and you combined. They will accuse you of lying, manipulating, being crazy and gaslight you and destroy your confidence especially when they tell you "I love you and you are best girlfriend ever on that day" and a year later "I never loved you and wanted to break up with you one month after meeting you" and you think "what the hell? How can someone be in relationship with me, live with me then change his mind because of what his friends say.

I knew all my life I was different and struggled to fit in socially. I also knew I always felt I had to survive alone as a lot of time no one was there to help me in the immediate moment I needed help. When I was 30, and after 2 years being on the waiting list, I was diagnosed with autistic spectrum disorder. I was diagnosed with generalised anxiety disorder a year later. Autism usually goes hand in hand with epilepsy. Reading more about it, I understood why I struggled with communicating effectively with people when conflicts arose, why I could not be diplomatic, why I struggled to feel comfortable in large crowds and could not understand jokes, or read between lines of what people said. I cannot distinguish when to be open with someone and who not to be open to and am overly trusting. This, in turn, has made people take advantage of me and use me in different ways.

My relationships have always been difficult although they always started well. I expected as someone with epilepsy to have a partner who understands my epilepsy and is not bothered by it nor does a runner, someone who has great empathy and vulnerability, someone who is happy to accompany me to hospitals and prioritise my medical needs when required above their social time, someone who does not tell me that I am "stupid" because of forgetting things that were said or appearing unremorseful due to not being able to recall certain events as result of many seizures; someone who loves me for who I am and accepts me, who is willing to look after my seizure alert dog when I go to hospital and who is willing to be a partner and family to me; someone who fully invests in me emotionally.

Sadly, I always struggled in relationships I have had and none of them had the fairytale ending although I almost had one this year which was the most special relationship to me and one that I truly felt would last.
The differences between our emotional growth and needs were too big despite me constantly trying to make the relationship work and holding it together. My health issues and the difference in communication language seemed to have gotten in the way.

Another issue I faced in my relationships is being too over giving and what I said was misinterpreted and misunderstood as I came across as difficult, sometimes called "crazy" and struggled to find balance and compromise.

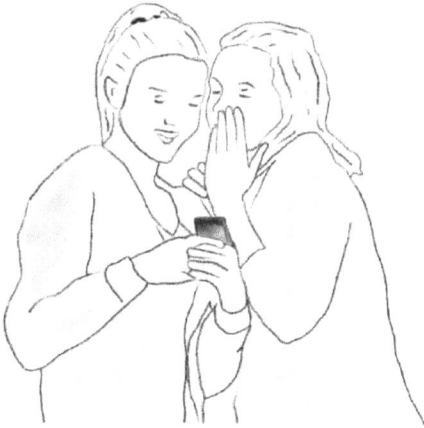

NEVER trust a "friend"
Who mixes with the ENEMY.

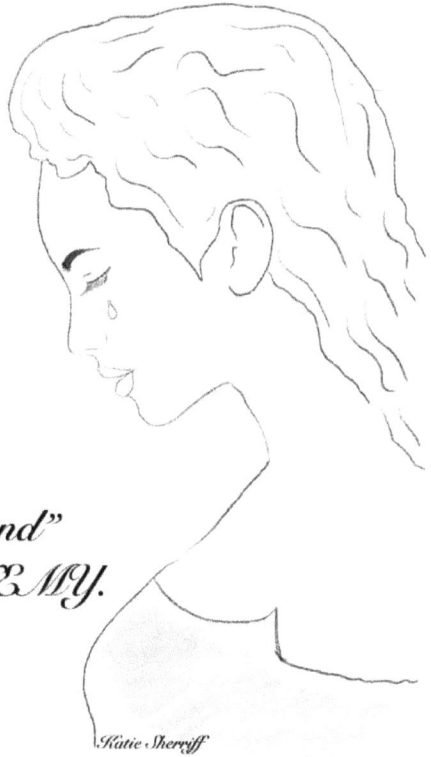

Katie Sherriff

Friend Issues When You Have Epilepsy

I have always struggled to make friends as people usually think I am strange, weird, psychotic or anti-social. However, a lot of people who do not know you, easily misjudge introverted people with invisible disabilities. In addition to this, if the person in question like myself, has been bullied or had bad experience, they will find it incredibly difficult to trust people they are not familiar with and therefore will be more suspicious of them and less willing to make friends. I have always been very introverted person and due to my autism and epilepsy combined with being bullied a lot, I have never been comfortable with having large group of friends. My belief was always to have small group of friends that you can trust rather than a large nest of acquaintances and two-faced friends who desert you at the first opportunity so as a result, I have always been extremely selective and put people through "friend interview stage" before allowing them to be my friends. I can frankly admit that I have made a lot of mistakes and trusted some people as friends who I should not have as they took advantage of me. I only had three true friends in primary and infant school, six true friends in secondary school, three true friends in college and two true friends at university. In workplaces I always either had only one friend or none at all as I never wanted to mix workplace with friendships and socializing in case I trusted too much and they took advantage of me to save their own skin which has happened to me at work a few times.

During school, I was severely bullied by both girls and boys and it made me afraid to make friends and trust people. At college, people would pretend to be friends with me until I did their homework and then shun me. At university, girls would take advantage of me financially by taking my money and manipulating me and gaslighting me because they knew I was desperate to have friends. At university no one wanted to work with me in groups and the lecturers always had to put me in groups with people who didn't want me in their group. I met my first two university friends in drama society and we have been friends ever since.

After university and in recent years I can safely say I feel I only have about five true friends who I can rely on through thick and thin and who know I will always be there for them no matter what. They know I will never let them down and know that I can safely say that they have always been there when I needed them most when no one else was there for me. I can safely say if it wasn't for Carolyn, Dom, Mandy, Lucy and Grace, I do not think I would have gotten out of my black hole and depression from a mixture of family bereavement, breakups, deteriorated health and increase in seizures and frustration at being misunderstood by society. Grace and Carolyn and Dom helped me in particular by teaching me to express my feelings through creative songwriting, singing, story writing and artwork. I feel if it wasn't for them, I would have exploded with anxiety, frustration and would be so depressed that I would have committed suicide when I felt everything was going wrong for me no matter how hard I tried and felt like everyone was dying around me, no one wanted to give me a chance and no one cared about me. These lovely angelic friends pulled me out of the black hole when doctors, nurses, counsellors and family could not because these people understood me and the anxiety, depression and bereavement I was going through when no one else did. Carolyn and Dom have been the strongest rocks for me and like unbreakable diamonds. Their empathy, gentleness, loving, supportive, understanding characters have meant the world to me and whenever I am with them along with Grace, I feel happiness and have massive smile on my face all the time and trust them with my life as opposed to being guarded, cautious and in warrior mode, constantly analysing situations and people.

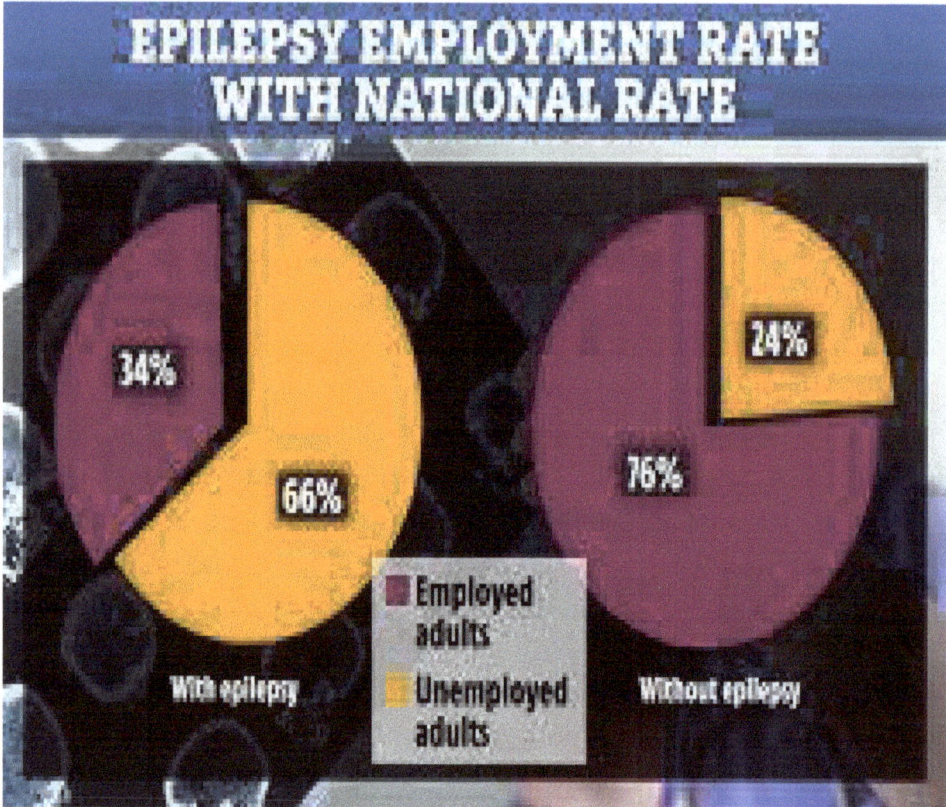

Epilepsy and Employment Issues so Employers Can Actually Understand You Instead of Overlooking You

In general, people find it relatively easy to find employment—either because they know people in the sector, because they are wealthy or because the jobs are handed to them on a silver plate. Disabled people, however, and epileptics in particular, find it not only difficult to find employment despite completing education and obtaining degrees, but also face discrimination in job specifications. While companies claim to be "disability confident" and "not discriminate against race, gender, disability, and age," this is simply not the case. Most job descriptions still contain clauses like "we are disability confident," yet specify that the job requires a driving license, for example. This is not being disability confident, as under DVLA rules, epileptics are not allowed to drive.

Other discriminatory examples on job adverts include requirements like having a 2:1 or above in your degree or attending a Russell Group University. Sadly, many working-class and disabled individuals cannot afford to attend Oxford or Cambridge University due to high fees, so they have to opt for non-Russell Group Universities. Some jobs claim not to discriminate on age, gender, looks, or disability, but this is often not true. For instance, police and forensic jobs are refused to individuals who do not pass their vision or fitness tests. Epileptics, in particular, have to look for local jobs because they are unable to drive, and public transport is often unreliable. This makes it even more difficult, as employers may prefer to hire a non-disabled person, even if they are less qualified than a disabled candidate.

Epileptics want to work, and they are often highly qualified in the sectors they studied for. They have the motivation, but it is heartbreaking to face so many rejections and be seen as unreliable due to their seizures, rather than being given the opportunity to work with reasonable adjustments. I have personally been fired from teaching for having seizures at work, despite requesting the adjustment of having a teaching assistant in my classroom who is trained in first aid to help and calm students down. This discrimination forces epileptics to apply for twice as many jobs, which undermines their confidence and leaves them feeling distrustful.

Employers need to change their job specifications and gain a better understanding of disabilities before claiming to be disability confident. Job descriptions need to be more flexible, and employers should engage with people with epilepsy to discuss improvements, instead of sticking to the same specifications that make it almost impossible for disabled people to have a future in employment. I have had to go through various jobs, but unfortunately, seizures and workplace bullying—often exacerbated by senior colleagues who felt threatened by my abilities—forced me out. Most of the time, I was so good at my job that my colleagues got jealous and tried to take credit for my work.

It is important for epileptics to get medical letters and have thorough discussions with employers about their condition and what adjustments can be made to help them. It is tragic that many epileptics cannot work in the sectors they are trained for because employers run for the hills or fail to offer proper accommodations. Moreover, many employers do not offer enough pay, which is a significant problem given the high medical costs epileptics face. As a result, epileptics are forced to find jobs that pay above the national minimum wage and are often full-time, due to the high current costs of living.

This situation causes a great deal of stress, but we have no choice but to cope. Employers need to recognize that epileptics are not unreliable for needing time off after a seizure, while we recover. Some people with epilepsy are entirely dependent on benefits, but with the latest government policies being discriminatory toward the disabled, it has become increasingly difficult to find jobs. Every job, no matter how basic or advanced, carries risks. For example, working in a pub and having a seizure could result in broken glass and injury. Similarly, working in haematology could pose a risk of incorrectly inserting a needle into a patient. Even in seemingly safe jobs like working in a library or as a hairdresser, a seizure could result in injury to oneself or others.

This is why it is vital for epileptics to explain their condition to employers, discuss potential risks, and outline the adjustments that can be made to ensure their safety at work. It is also important to join a union to protect against discrimination. After working in many jobs, I have come to realize that a public workplace is not for me due to the stress of competing with numerous job applicants. I have decided to pursue courses that will allow me to work from home, where I can set my own schedule. I can write books, proofread, and translate, instead of constantly being scrutinized and rejected by those higher up, who are often lazy and take credit for my hard work.

Of course, working from home is not for everyone, but for epileptics, it can be a way to reduce the stress and anxiety that traditional workplaces bring. This is especially true until employers complete proper training on epilepsy and make changes to job descriptions to be more inclusive and less discriminatory toward epileptics.

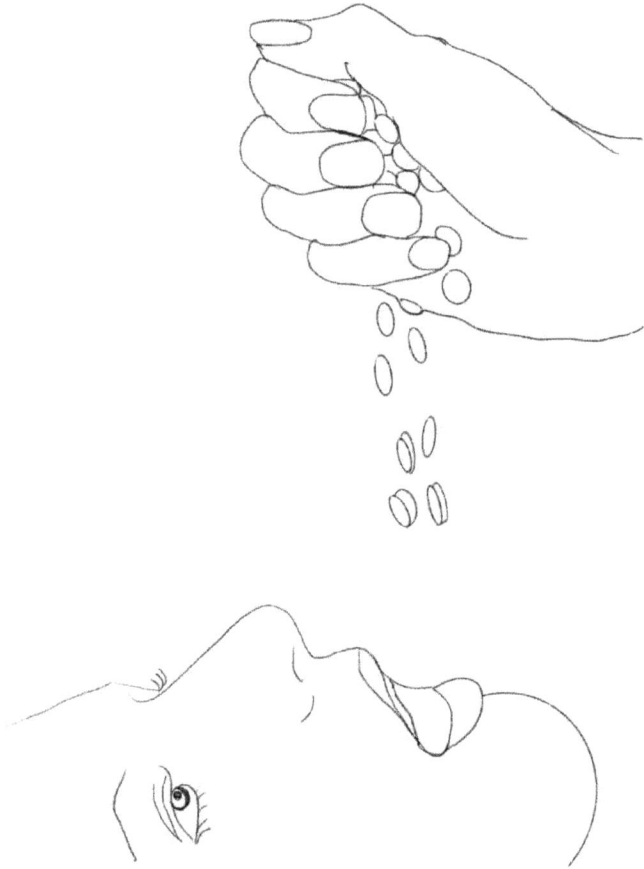

Trouble With DWP and Benefits and How To Win Pip Tribunal Appeals

It is a very sorry state we live in today's society. People who genuinely have had and still have long-term disabilities and mental health issues find it difficult and frustrating that they are not believed and are treated like lying scum by the DWP (Department for Work and Pensions) for being honest. They have to prove their disability every year to the DWP to keep their disability benefits. Meanwhile, some the former DWP bosses, (now replaced by someone with the same mentality), and all the people who work there, are liars themselves and thieves. The disabled people who have to jump through hoops to keep their benefits and prove constantly their medical condition that they are not liars and are not fraudsters nor steal or ruin people's lives. It is the DWP that ruins people's lives and ways of living, while not caring if the disabled candidates live or die, as long as they get their chunky pay check for denying benefits. They get upset if the disabled candidates beat them in court and call them out on their wrongdoings, as I have done every few years.

Despite extensive medical evidence from top neurologists, GPs, and other medical professionals, the DWP assessors often think they know better than the top neurologists who have treated patients for over 20 years. Most of the time, the DWP assessors are not even qualified neurologists. They may be social workers, dentists, or have qualifications in fields totally unrelated to the specific condition or disability. Majority of people with disabilities have higher costs of living due to the costs of their medications, constant hospital visits, and needing to pay to get to places because they cannot drive. They cannot afford rent and bills without benefits due to their disabilities being so severe that they cannot work. Some people also have to pay for blue badges and mobility scooters if they have a high enough PIP (Personal Independence Payment) score. All of this costs more than someone who is not disabled.

Epileptic medications are some of the most expensive medications and can also be some of the most dangerous due to the effects they have on the brain. There is also a need to be careful with dosages, and patients can only get a certain amount per month on repeat prescriptions. The DWP will do everything to reject an application, not believe the applicant, and make them go through an appeal, mandatory reconsideration, and then face them in person at a tribunal in court just to be able to get the disability benefits they deserve. I fight every year for myself and other epileptics against the DWP because I feel we do not deserve to be put under stress deliberately, especially when the DWP knows from medical evidence that stress is a major trigger for seizures. We are not circus animals or scammers lying about our conditions to get disability benefits. It is shameful that we need to prove our condition and not be believed by the DWP, most of whose staff have no common sense or knowledge of neurological disabilities. They think epilepsy goes away within a week, like the flu, when it does not.

When I question their knowledge of epilepsy in court and ask them how they would feel if I made them prove their medical condition every year, did not believe medical professionals, and the person who has had the disability for years, they usually have no answer. When you test them on their epilepsy knowledge, they either do not answer or try to change the subject because they know they were wrong. You have to play a psychological game with the DWP and guilt-trip them into understanding how they would feel if the shoe were on the other foot, if they were the disabled applicant and not believed. You must make them jump through hoops and give them a taste of their own medicine, or else you will never get the benefits that are rightfully yours. You have to convince the court of the DWP's lack of knowledge on your condition and how they always misjudge and mis-assess you because they are arrogant and believe they know better than the top neurologists who have been in charge of your condition for over 20 years. You have to name and shame them to bring their egos down and make them realize they are not invincible. Just because you have an invisible illness does not give them the right to bully, psychologically abuse, and make you prove everything to them while they have no medical knowledge or common sense.

It is like giving a housefly the position to judge whether someone is disabled—that is the amount of knowledge the DWP has about your condition. The key is to fight with everything you have and to never give up. They never want to lose against you because it means a dent in their pay check, and they do not wish to ruin their reputation and image further. The more you stand up to the DWP, the better it is for you. It is always a very long stressful and drawn out battle as the DWP does everything to make you psychologically stressed and to try to make you give up. The judge and jury will always be understanding of your condition and look more favourably upon you, your struggles with the condition, and the effort you made to gather all the evidence needed in your fight to be believed for telling the truth.

As of 2023, the guidelines and laws regarding the DWP changed. I received a back payment, as did everyone else with epilepsy and other disabilities, due to the inability to attend DWP assessments during the pandemic. Thanks to the work of the Epilepsy Society, Scope, Professor Sander, and other neurologists, along with the hard battle of disabled people, the government had to bow to pressure and disclose to the public how many assessments they failed to win due to incompetence. Previously, the law was changed by former government minister so that there will no longer be DWP assessments for disabled people with a long-term health condition or incurable disability that prevents them from being able to work or live their life properly. This was a huge positive change by him as it minimises a lot of stress with the assessments for people with epilepsy who feel they need to jump rings in a circus to prove their medical condition every few years for a condition they have for life most of the time.

I had to battle against Compare the Market after their advert contained several severe flashing lights and a meerkat choking. I reported it to the Advertising Standards Agency, Channel 4, and won after they acknowledged that the advert breached guidelines by not letting people know it contained severe flashing lights, which can trigger epileptics, as well as people with eating disorders and mental health issues. Since then, that particular advert was replaced with a new one that does not feature flashing lights or show someone having an allergic reaction. However, I have recently noticed that the flashy Compare the Meerkat advert has been put back up on Channel 4, 5, and Pluto TV for Halloween and Christmas, showing that they have no regard for epileptics or for Zach's Law, or for laws in general. I feel there needs to be a giant petition to get this advert banned, as it poses a danger to all photosensitive people, epileptics, and those with neurological conditions. The advert gives no warning of how flashy it is and puts people in danger of seizures. The TV companies need to be fined hugely to learn their lesson and compensate every epileptic for endangering their lives with adverts that we cannot avoid whenever we wish to watch TV.

In the most recent government, the new DWP chief thinks it is fantastic idea to invade financial privacy of disabled people. This bill was discussed but not passed fully in October 2024 due to numerous concerns about privacy. it was later passed which allows the DWP to invade financial privacy of disabled people and take their money and cut benefits as they see it as fraud even though they know PIP is not income. I disputed this as fraud and not following own policies about benefit cap not applying to those on limited capability to work and on PIP which is not means tested. They are delaying my PIP tribunal as they know they breached their own policies and making disabled suffer financially, medically and psychologically by refusing to give evidence at tribunals and delaying mandatory reconsideration for over 10 weeks. This has breached the Fraud Act by stealing non means tested PIP money from disabled. This is a disgraceful bill which many companies and charities as well as public have protested and is invasion of human rights, however DWP are ignoring this and the only way this will be overturned is with the help of European court of Human Rights. The DWP believe a disabled person can live on 6k a year- when rent and bills alone are at least 1k for non-disabled and 2k or more for disabled without food costs which for disabled people cost more. Disabled people cannot rely on foodbanks as people with epilepsy in particular usually have food sensitivities. I have to rely on ketogenic diet, cannot have salt and high carb foods and so cannot rely on foodbanks as a lot of tinned foods in food banks are high carb and high salt or high sugar in order to preserve their shelf life and make the food last longer. The real fraudsters are top government officials, DWP and MPs who are the REAL tax avoiders! They are the ones who should be living on bare minimum and made to pay back all the tax avoidance money and give homes they do not use back to the public. It is important to research all DWP laws and remember that DWP are disability bullies who do not care about you and take pleasure in torturing the disabled and stressing them out unfairly whilst making them live in poverty. they are responsible for many disability and welfare suicides and records show it. The key to defeating them each time is to research all their laws and fight against their discrimination towards you, point out their mistakes and what the laws are and play human chess with them- ensure you checkmate them into a corner and remind them that no one is above the law. The reason they do not care about discriminating you and take pleasure is because they still get their paycheque at end of day regardless of discrimination which is wrong- I have fought them for years and they are not great at listening nor good at following their own laws- most of them have an attitude of " do what I say or be penalised" but they are cowards when you stand up to them like bullies in playground and would hate being put in your predicament and living situation and you need to use this as a weapon against them as this always works to your advantage. Also as they are not very bright, but rely solely on gift of the gab, use legal knowledge against them- it always works.

Adult Years and Epilepsy

Epilepsy can change at any point in life—sometimes it can worsen, and the seizures become more frequent and more aggressive, and with other people, seizures can improve and become less frequent and less violent. In others, epileptic seizures can stay the same.

My epilepsy as a child started as convulsions, and I struggled to walk until the medication was changed and then they turned into absence seizures throughout childhood. However, my seizures turned for the worse into drug-resistant grand mal epilepsy in 2007 following the stress of being dismissed unfairly from a job and a bad reaction to having a defibrillator put in, following collapsing and being diagnosed with tachycardia (overly fast heart rate). The defibrillator caused my brain and body to have too much electricity, and therefore my epilepsy changed from absences to grand mal seizures.

I also found out at this time that I have a serious allergy to codeine after being given it post-op, and my throat closed up. They had to give me anti-allergy medication and unblock my throat. At this time, I became resistant every few months to every anti-epileptic medication I took, which became a nightmare for my neurologist and also a very confusing and complex issue. I developed generalized anxiety disorder shortly after my loss of job, and each time I had a stressful and traumatic experience, be it relationship-related, job-related, DWP-related, or education-related, it made the anxiety worse, and I have needed counselling, but the waiting lists have been very long. The counselling has helped a lot, but I still have anxiety.

I was diagnosed with autism in 2018, which made anxiety and seizures worse with a fear of large crowds. I had to face my fear throughout university and completed two degrees at the same time, along with being part of the drama society, as well as doing post-graduation, working as a radiologist in Middlesbrough, teacher training in Watford, proofreading and translation in London, and then working in various schools throughout London and Hertfordshire before working as a lecturer in college, where I rose to the position of course leader to teach not just biology, but also chemistry, physics, access to science and health professions, and forensic science.

It was overwhelming, all the teachings, marking, lesson planning, pastoral responsibilities, teacher training, and traveling several hours from Watford to Weybridge and back every day. My father died of cancer while I was working, and I had a seizure at work, lost my temporary home in Weybridge, and had a mental breakdown. One of my students and her parent took pity on me and asked me to stay the night over on her parent's sofa, to which I agreed as I was feeling bad post-seizure and mental breakdown and over-exhausted to travel four hours back home. But the parent told my workplace, and I got fired for having a seizure at work, then not traveling back to Watford when I was in a confused state post-seizure.

I worked in other schools after this but never got a high position as this again. I had to deal with bad relationships, domestic abuse, numerous pregnancies and abortions, friend betrayals, bullying, abandonment, homewreckers, and backstabbers and learned to trust and rely only on myself. I gained my living independence and moved away from living with my mum in 2016 on my birthday after being on the waiting list for 10 years. At this time, I got my seizure alert dog, Chess, from the Dogs Trust. He was very anxious and nervous as a puppy, but after completing puppy skills, puppy socialization, and obedience with Dogs Trust, I got first behaviourist Heather Wren at Dogs Trust to help me with recall, and then I got help from Assistance Dogs and behaviourist Ashleigh to help me with seizure alert training, which he did brilliantly.

He settled into the home really well and has become not only my lifeline and helper but also family. He has won 8 medals, including Best in Show and Reserve Best in Show and Best Rescue. He is so friendly with everyone and has been taught to bark loudly when he sees me having a seizure for help. He is not aggressive but does love to hug everyone he meets, and he has helped not only my epilepsy but also my autistic social anxiety too, as I feel less fearful when walking with him than being around others alone and fearing having a seizure around them.

After this, I did several jobs which were paid, but they never lasted very long, along with volunteering which lasted several years but sadly was never paid. I have done also several courses, but sadly long-term well-paid jobs I can be in for many years seem to evade me. I have created this book and am thrilled that finally, someone realizes, appreciates, and loves the passion, heart, soul, courage, and hard work I have put in to raise awareness and improve the lives of others like me with the condition, as well as help their friends, families, employers, and the unintelligent, unemphatic government understand the condition and understand humanity.

I was originally also thrilled that finally I found my soulmate, who understands my autism, my epilepsy, and accepts my seizures and deals with my anxiety, whilst I deal with his ADHD, and I finally feel happy and safe at being cared for rather than abandoned or punched and left to cope alone with the aftermath. Although having to deal with most things alone and organizing everything alone is still very stressful and frustrating. Sadly my soulmate ran away from me believing I was the problem which I wasn't and it hurt so much. I hope he realizes the truth one day he was lied to by people jealous of me to believe things about me that were not true.

You really have to fight hard in this life—you will be broken several times, but you have to rise like a phoenix from the ashes and not let anyone or anything get in the way of what you wish to achieve—no matter how hard it is. Do not settle for less than your worth and be proud every day of who you are and what you have achieved so far.

THE EPILEPTIC WARRIOR PRINCESS

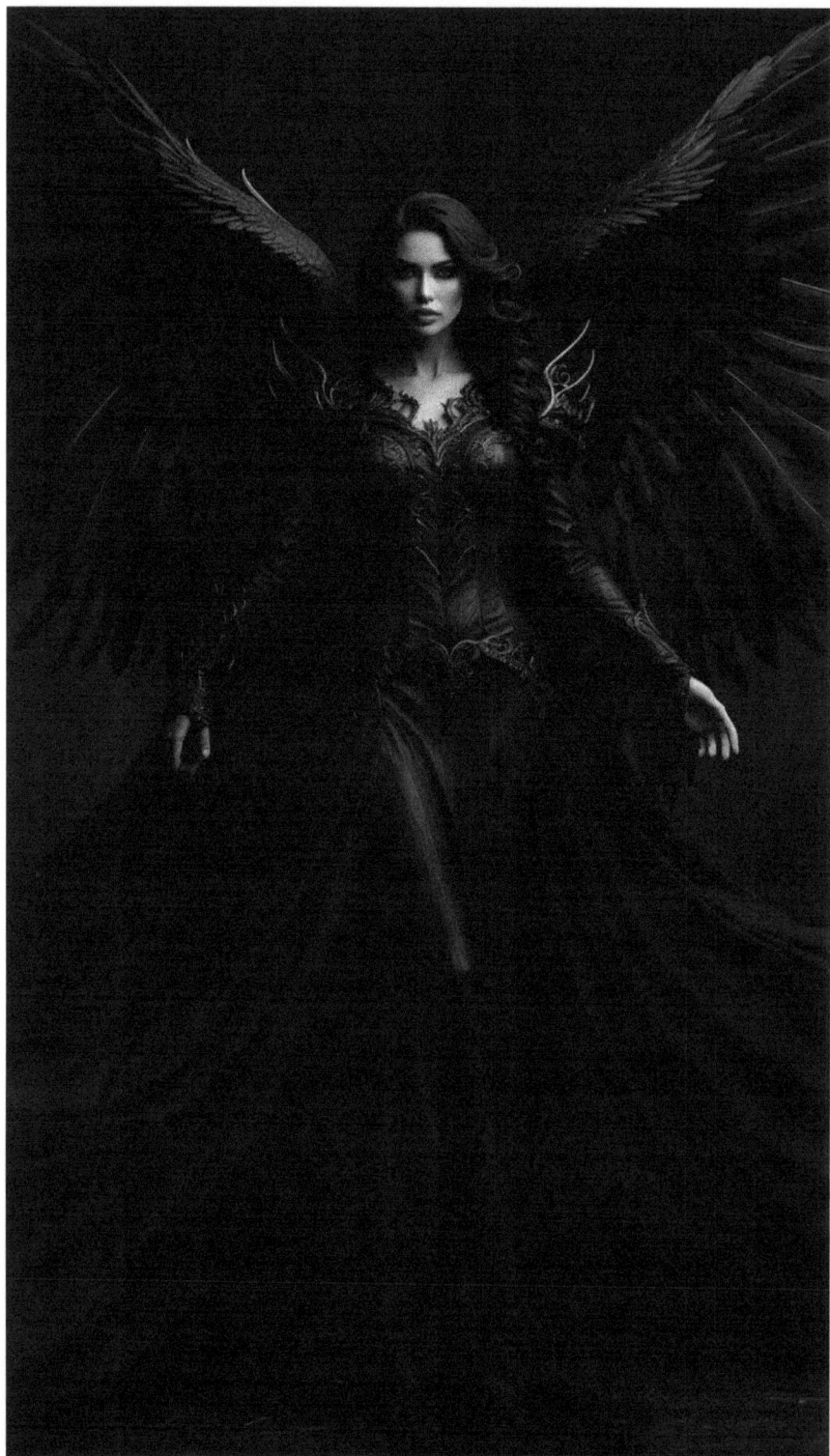

How To Cope with Death of Family Members and Other Stressful Situations and Overcome Them

This is one of the hardest topics to deal with when you have epilepsy, but particularly if you had a strong bond with the family member. People with epilepsy do not cope well with highly emotional situations and stressful situations as stress is a major trigger for seizures.

I myself have had to learn through different tried and tested methods that the best way to cope with death of a family member is to keep their memory alive and keep a part of them such as photos of them close to me whilst accepting their death. My nutty gran's death was the hardest for me as I was extremely close to my nutty granny and she taught me a lot of subjects from learning how to cook, to teaching me languages when I was super young, to making reading books exciting, teaching me poetry, teaching me how to be charming but witty. Not accepting that they have died makes you feel overwhelmed and always living in false hope which is never a good thing- for the first two years after nutty granny passed away, I kept hoping her death wasn't real, but the more I kept hoping, the more stressed and disappointed I got when I faced reality and knew she wasn't alive anymore.

Other stressful situations such as job interviews-make sure you learn everything about the company, make sure you have all the qualifications, do not go into an interview like an airhead but be polite, and do not let HR take advantage of you-they will look for any excuse to not employ you because of your disability. Ask them everything at the interview-if they want to know everything about you, put them in situation where they have to answer scenarios what they would do so you get a feel about working alongside them and where you are able to get to know the type of people they are. HR are not kind- they are the employment DWP who will look for any loophole to not employ you or to get rid of you, so find out everything about them and the company and do not trust them because they never have your best interests at heart.

It is important when faced with stressful situations that you face your bullies head on-deep inside they are weak insecure individuals who like to feel big by preying on people they believe are weaker than themselves. This is why I have always stood up not only for myself but for whole of epilepsy patients against the bullying staff in Chalfont especially the receptionist who kept bullying me constantly (mostly due to jealousy that she was getting fat and old) by telling me "stop breathing", "stop speaking" " stop laughing" but retreating when I stood up for myself and other patients to her and told her to put some appropriate clothes on instead of dressing like dragon from Shrek going to a Britney concert whilst undergoing medication changes and told her she is neither my mother nor my neurologist to tell me what to do and if she had sense she would dress appropriately for a hospital and show respect to patients instead of being a bully if she wants to keep her job, stood up for other people including my partner, stood up against homewreckers and even took them to court, stood up against HR and DWP and always put people in their place who tried to put me down and blame me for their job and life faults. I have always appeared intimidating and although not won every battle against them, it has changed the way people see things and made them learn and change their mentality towards disabled people and to not be so narrow minded.

How To Help Medical Staff at Hospital Understand Your Condition Better (Even If You Are the Most Complex Patient They Have)

Doctors and neurologists go by what they learn in their medical degrees and books but applying this to patients in daily life is another story as every patient has unique DNA and therefore will react very differently to each medication and dosage they are given. If the patient in addition has other underlying health conditions, you must let neurologist and nurses and doctors know as other medications can affect the effects of anti-epileptic medication and sometimes other medications do not mix well with anti-epileptic medications so doctors and all medical professionals need to know all your medical conditions to be able to work with all your conditions, other medical professionals if you have other underlying conditions and see what medications can work alongside each other without side effects whilst improving your epilepsy and other underlying health issues that you may have e.g. I have to take bisoprolol for arrythmia for the heart alongside my antiepileptic medication but there is no medication for autism except trying to learn to cope with situations I find difficult such as social situations, trying to learn to be more diplomatic and attempting to make new friends which is difficult due to trust issues.

I have the most amazing neurologist in Professor Sander at National Hospital for Neurology and Neurosurgery who I have had as my neurologist for 22 years and he has never given up on me. He refuses to retire until he can solve the mystery of my seizures as I am his most complex patient. We have gone through loads of different medications but I am so proud that he refuses to give up on me and carries the journey on with me instead of seeing me as a hopeless case who will never stop the seizure. I have always done my best to help from my end with keeping seizure diary and detailing how each medication makes me feel at each appointment. I have had a rare time where I have been seizure free for maximum of three months and told Professor Sander that I believe the dosages are right but also that seizures improved since defibrillator was turned off at St Barts as there is less electricity in my body and brain and I believe this has helped medically him too learn about how different organs such as the heart can have an impact on the brain and epilepsy as result of the electrical impulses going through the nerves within the body. I have also let him know that I have had less emotional stress this year and this has been a big part of my epilepsy and seizures decreasing as I am not feeling overly stressed out and panicky all the time although I do still have anxiety for life which he understands and has written in his medical letters, and as a result, I am having help for this to decrease stress and anxiety whilst taking medication regularly. For me, I could not have a better neurologist and it is so important to have a neurologist who you feel listens to you and understand you and is honest with you about your condition even it seems harsh at times. It is important to know the truth and ask all questions- do not feel like you are being a waste of time, but ask anything you are worried or do not know about relating to your condition during your appointment as appointments are usually once a year and you get a limited amount of time with the neurologist due to their busy schedules. I would gladly be happy if Professor Sander won award for best neurologist and for his contribution to epilepsy research and epilepsy society. I hope he never retires.

I also have had the most amazing GP in Dr Anne Anderson who has always taken care of me, listened to me, referred me to support systems I needed such as counselling and physio, always made sure I have enough medication on time as repeat prescriptions and always made me feel comfortable describing my issues and asking questions about my health and going to appointments. She is my favourite GP who has always shown and given her time to her patients along with loyalty and respect and has the greatest empathy of any GP I have known and seen. She taught me to never give up hope when I felt my health was rock bottom and always cracked jokes to make me feel better about my health in my appointment visits. I always have felt I could trust her and Professor Sander with my life when trust is not easy for me to come by. I hope she never retires as it would be great loss for me.

How to Help Parents When You Have Epilepsy

It is difficult for any parent to raise a child—especially if they are a single parent, as it is a change of lifestyle, change in financial circumstances, change in emotional and psychological state, and change in career and relationships. It is even harder when your child has epilepsy as a baby or young child, or develops it while they are growing up. Please be aware that it is a learning curve for both yourself as a parent and for your child learning to live and cope with the condition. It will be a stressful and emotional journey for both parent and child. However, it is vital that communication is good between parent and child, bond and relations are good, and that the parent is supportive on all levels—from helping get support for epilepsy, helping get medication regularly, supervising the child when showering, ensuring certain sports such as wrestling with others are banned due to possible further head injuries, that the child communicates how they feel, parent calls for help and attends neurology appointments when required, as well as calling the neurologist for advice.

It is important the parent learns basic first aid for when seizures occur to help the child restart breathing correctly and look after them until they fully recover and their memory returns. It is vital for the child to maintain inside themselves a strong will and to never give up on anything in life— never give up on themselves, hopes and dreams, and never give up on their self-esteem. Most importantly, fight for everything you believe in. Say this saying to yourself daily: "If I do not believe in myself and the things I can achieve, why should anyone else believe in me? It starts with me—I believe in myself and I will achieve whatever I put my mind to, no matter how long it takes or how many attempts it takes."

You are responsible for your health, especially as you get older, while your parent is responsible for your health during your early years, but never feel sorry for your child—it is a bump throughout life and a part of them. Take the rocky road, treat your child like normal, despite seizures here and there, and encourage them that they are as able to succeed as those without the condition. Encourage, inspire, and boost their self-belief.

My mum was my rock throughout my life. She helped me when I developed my epilepsy at the age of 2 after a bad reaction to the MMR vaccine, which originally gave me a high temperature but then progressed to convulsions, and I was diagnosed with epilepsy. She has helped me gain my medication regularly and the repeat prescriptions throughout childhood, as well as helped me throughout the PIP appeals, which are very stressful, as well as teaching me how to maintain stress levels throughout school when I felt very stressed with the amount of homework, as well as how no one wanted me in their teams and how I felt lonely throughout a lot of my life, except when I had the people I loved and who mattered the most close to me, whether they were family, friends, or my favourite teacher.

I had to learn to stand on my own two feet and learn a lot of things alone without help, and this has helped me throughout life to learn independence from a young age and not to rely on many people, but as the saying goes, "If you want something done right, you do it yourself," although your parent can help you in the early years while you are very young. Everybody makes mistakes in life and no one gets absolutely everything correct the first time, so do not feel ashamed or embarrassed about making mistakes or not knowing what to do in situations you have never encountered before. Support your parent and appreciate everything they do for you and have done for you—once they are gone, no one can replace the love and support you received from them, especially in the hardest times.

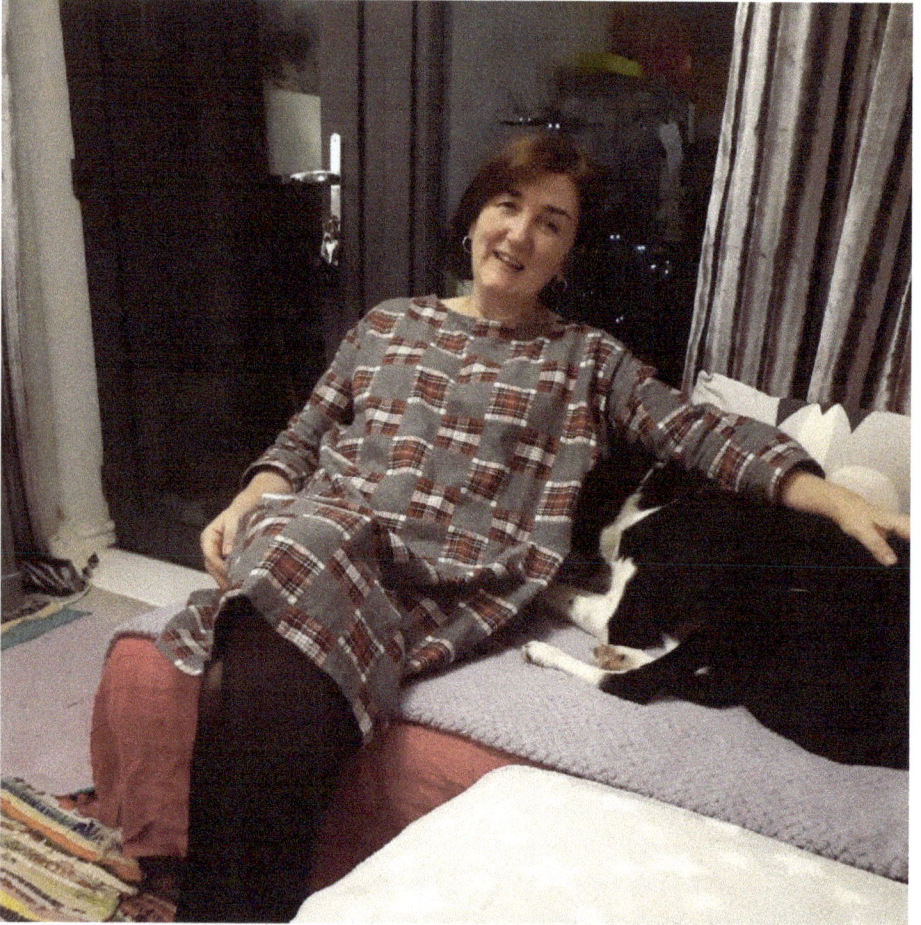

My lovely supportive mum with my lovely seizure alert dog Chess who both have been my rock.

How to Cope When You Feel Overwhelmed

The best things to do when you feel overwhelmed are:

Walks in the park for about an hour or so-either alone or with the dog

Doing some artwork to express how you feel or writing poems describing your feelings

Do a little bit of housework at a time to feel relief, lower stress and feel sense of achievement-do not do too much at once to avoid feeling tired and overwhelmed too quickly

Talk to a charity such as Epilepsy Society, Herts Mind Network and reach out to supportive friends who will listen to you when you need it most

Do enjoyable hobbies you enjoy- be it painting, playing board games, learning new skills- I love learning new languages, dancing and reading as well as inventing my own cooking recipes as I find baking therapeutic.

Treat yourself to a massage once or twice a month to ease tension in areas of the body and head you feel stressed in.

THE EPILEPTIC WARRIOR PRINCESS

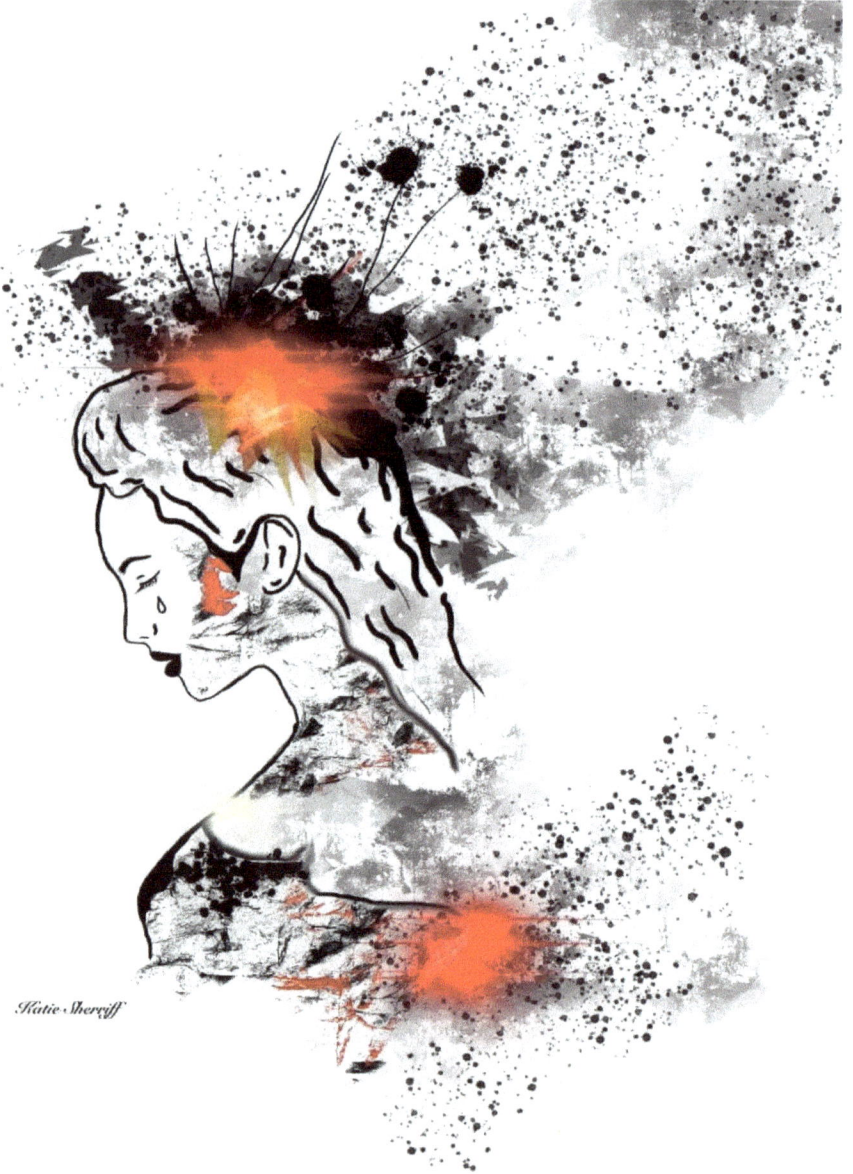

Katie Sherriff

Things to Do to Help Seizures Become More Controlled and How to Try to Get Seizure Free

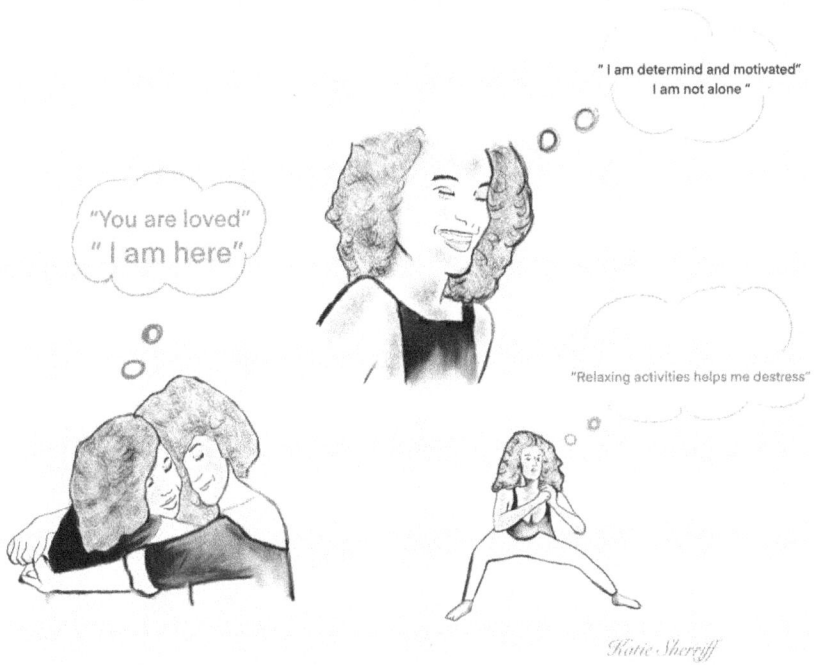

Medication does not always control seizures fully and majority of people will be on anti-epileptic medication for life. It is therefore important to be able to do certain things that minimize the triggers and help your seizures become more controlled in the hope that eventually the person can become seizure free. If you are a family member, friend or partner of someone with epilepsy, here are a few things you can do to help their seizures become more controlled without their medication:

- Do relaxing activities together that helps them destress as stress is one of the main triggers for all epileptics- whether this is drawing together, singing together, going for a relaxing walk or other form of exercise such as dance classes, yoga
- Encourage and motivate them so they do not feel like a failure and isolated all the time
- Offer them emotional support-this is a major one, because if we feel overwhelmed and alone with no one to talk to, our brains go into overanalytical mode to try to solve the issue ourselves and it turns usually into a vicious stressful circle with no resolution. However, if someone is there for us and prepared to listen to us and offer their advice or just be someone we can talk to, we feel less stressed and with decreased stress levels, we are less likely to have a seizure as well as be more trusting of people.
- Remind us to take our medication-sometimes due to having seizures, post seizure we cannot remember if we have taken our medication or not and need to set alarms when to take our medications or someone to tell us if we have taken it or not due to our temporary memory loss. Please do not feel embarrassed or afraid to tell us as we would rather appreciate you telling us truthfully that we forgot to take our medication by accident than us overdosing by taking too much of our medication due to us not remembering taking our medication.
- Call an ambulance if you see us seizuring instead of panicking and running away- I know it is not a pretty sight seeing someone having a seizure, but we would appreciate it more if you moved dangerous things out of the way to avoid less injury during

seizure and called for help if you see a person having a seizure than panicking and running away and leaving them to fend for themselves on the floor or in the street or wherever they are having a seizure. Also time the length of the seizure as paramedics and doctors will ask you this and we cannot know this whilst seizuring so are usually unable to answer this question and rely on others to tell our doctors this.

Things You Are Restricted to And Cannot Do with Uncontrolled Epilepsy That Others Overlook and Take for Granted

Due to the fact that there are many different types of epilepsy, in this chapter I will be listing only the ones that apply to my epilepsy and how it restricts my life. Some people may be able to relate to this whilst others will not relate to it due to having different form of epilepsy or not having it at all

Here are some of the things that drug-resistant tonic-clonic epilepsy with eyelid myoclonia restricts you to:

- Not being able to drive-limits you jobwise as you cannot apply for jobs that require driving license and have to rely on public transport to get everywhere which isn't always reliable. You cannot get a job just anywhere as you rely on public transport and job requires you to be there usually for 8.30am or 9am so if the public transport takes over 1hr to get to your destination and buses run every hour, you are better off only looking locally which means you cannot always apply for job related to your degree or try to get your dream job.
- Not able to shower or take baths alone- due to unpredictable seizures and risk of concussion or drowning or both. This means someone must always supervise you in case you have a seizure which can feel embarrassing and awkward having a seizure whilst naked for both you and person supervising you. It can be more difficult when you are on holiday due to not always being able to be in the bathroom with you due to the space or you travelling alone.
- Not able to handle flashing lights and having to wear super dark sunglasses everywhere night and day. This makes it difficult when your partner and his friends are musicians to see them because you cannot see anything through your sunglasses but can

hear them and if you take sunglasses off, you risk having seizure. It is also a problem with going to cinemas, theatres and certain TV adverts and programmes such as Eurovision which do not give clear warnings beforehand nor make programme suitable and safe for epileptics. I also cannot watch fireworks as they set off my seizures.

- Stress- most people can handle a bit of stress and do not have a seizure when stressed or overwhelmed. I, however, have seizures when overstressed and overwhelmed which makes everything difficult because everything in life is stressful. I constantly have to try to reduce my stress levels to avoid having seizures.

- Communication with people- after a seizure I am usually very confused and the more someone tries to get me to talk whilst severely confused, the more frustrated in myself I get because until I recover from seizure my memory is usually very poor and I have no recollection of events or what I am saying. For people who do not know me well, they either think I am stupid, playing stupid or being mean and it turns usually into a vicious cycle of frustration as I feel like I am constantly misjudged and misunderstood.

- Difficulty talking about condition to people- I find it difficult due to mixture of memory loss, anxiety and not being able to trust people to talk to people about my condition due to the fact I was not believed constantly by employers and DWP even with medical evidence from my neurologist and constantly had to fight for justice and to be treated right. As a result, I do not feel able to talk to employers, people I meet or anyone and feel forced to tell DWP about my condition even though I know they deliberately reject me to put me through stress knowing it is a trigger for me and want me to fight them.

- Not able to get jobs you like-epilepsy hinders you to get jobs you like because employers deem you a medical burden or risk even if you have the qualifications and skills they require for the job or even if you have a lot of experience, they overlook you for someone with no experience who has gift of the gab and no epilepsy or health issues. However usually people with epilepsy are not stupid or dumb like employers believe and have a more genius brain than someone without epilepsy. I have had to fight constantly to get a job and usually put HR people and employers in their place and make them realize they are being discriminatory towards people with invisible disabilities by not giving them jobs when they are capable of doing the job.

- Relationship and family issues- due to side effects of our medications, epileptics can sometimes have a horrendous and obsessively aggressive temper due to feeling frustrated and feeling that life isn't fair. We normally take it out on those closest to us because we feel misunderstood by the people, we are supposed to trust the most and those that are meant to know and understand us. This can lead to people abandoning us including family members, not just partners and feeling anxious, depressed, having abandonment and trust issues and being unable to open up to people due to fear. In addition, if we had deep-rooted family issues or traumatic events relating to people in the past, we will find talking and opening up even harder.

Why others overlook the condition in today's society!
"I believe awareness needs to be mandatory in workplace "

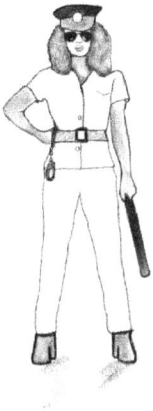

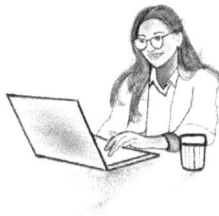

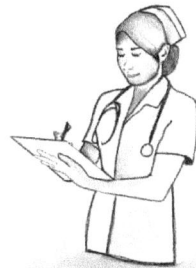

Katie Sherriff

Why Others Overlook the Condition in Today's Society

Sadly, whilst certain medical conditions such as blindness and deafness are talked about and teaching sign language to help deaf people and braille to help blind people as well as basic first aid in workplaces, majority of how to cope and deal with invisible disabilities such as epilepsy, hydrocephalus, ADHD, Autism, schizophrenia, bipolar disorder, multiple personality disorder, depression, anxiety disorders are not on the agenda in most workplaces and therefore majority of employers and employees have little to no knowledge of the conditions and how to deal with it until they experience it themselves.

Although recognition of some of the conditions is rising, invisible disabilities still remain widely unacknowledged in workplaces without people being taught how to cope with them. This makes it more difficult for people with the condition particularly if they have more than one condition alone such as myself with heart issues, epilepsy and anxiety disorder as work colleagues, employers, DWP and your partner's friends and family friends do not know how to cope or what to do if they see you having a seizure and do not know how to cope with someone having anxiety attack which looks similar to panic attack.

As a result, many epileptics with other health conditions such as depression or anxiety disorders feel isolated and ostracized due to no fault of their own. I believe more awareness needs to be made mandatory in workplace, the same way braille, sign language and safeguarding and basic first aid CPD courses are mandatory in most workplaces, the same should apply to invisible disabilities.

Currently in my experiences a lot of people do not believe I am epileptic because I am not in a wheelchair and my seizures happen at unpredictable times. Also there needs to be more knowledge of the conditions particularly with the DWP and PIP as assessors who do the assessments usually have no knowledge of the condition and life with the condition and make unfair assumptions and judgements.

The DWP have most recently been even more cruel towards people with disabilities alongside with the help of the new Prime Minister to allow DWP to invade disabled people's privacy and bank accounts because the DWP generalize and see cruelly that all disabled people are fraudsters which is not the case-Government people are fraudsters. Yet, because they know that disabled people do not have the financial means to fight back and are easily broken with being accused, they now threaten disabled people and invade their financial privacy and human rights.

This I consider illegal bill that has been passed and needs to be banned as myself and other disabled people have equal human rights as non disabled. We have rights to disability benefits if we rightfully with medical evidence shown have a lifelong condition and the DWP should not be probing our bank accounts nor making us prove our seizures every 3 years.

People also expect too much from you when your health cannot take it and dismiss you or do not give you a chance because they believe you cannot do the job or are not a nice person. People generally, although this does not apply to everyone, do not believe you are epileptic if they cannot see it and this is something that needs changing the views on.

Quotes I Live By in Life

"If you want something done right, youhave to do it yourself"

" If you do not belief in yourself, why should anyone else? "

"Trust in yourself and you can achieve anything"

"Failure is not an option"

"Not everyone is your friend"

"Do not give up on dreams and never giveup even during hardest times"

"Only keep friends who are there for you through hardest times as well as easy times- not the ones who only appear when they need something from you"

"Life is full of obstacles- treat everything like a battlefield"

"Do not jump rivers for people who will not jump puddles for you"

"Take responsibility for all choices you make as you are the one who has to live with them"

"Rely on no one but yourself and learn as much as you can alone"

"Try to not wear your heart on your sleeve-you never know who is holding a knife to stab you in the back"

" Be kind, respectful, honest, loving and understanding but try to not allow yourself to be used"

" Without hardship and struggle and heartbreak, you cannot gain wisdom, love and strength"

"Nobody knows absolutely everything- so do not allow anyone to put you down who has not lived your life nor been in your situation"

"Always stand up and fight for justice- no one has right to breach your human rights"

"Rules were created for the obedience of fools and the guidance of wise men- do not be a fool.

" Being nice gets you used- being wise gets you respected"

" Treat others the way you wish to be treated- if you mistreat me or my closest circle you will get burnt"

"Only the weak bully your closest allies and try to turn them against you because they are scared and intimidated by you"

"Do homework on your opponents first-do not charge into battle blind"

"The flower that blooms in austerity is the rarest and most beautiful of all"

"Write your own story, follow your heart, and find love in your own time. "

"You cannot turn back time and no one lives forever, so make decisions you feel are right for you, fight for what you believe to be true and right and do not regret any decisions you make as even bad decisions and choices are a lesson to be learnt from"

"Appreciate what others do for you- its not often that people show appreciation and care" and thank them and show appreciation in return.

"What we do in life, echoes in eternity"

THE EPILEPTIC WARRIOR PRINCESS

"Do not care what people think- those who like you will stand by you- those who hate you or dislike you are not worth your time, energy or effort but so what!"

"Do not settle for less than what you are worth and always reach for the top"

"You need to grow in orderto know, you need to learn in order to earn and you need to read in order to lead"

"Never forget the hand who put you where you were- lots of bosses and politicians forget it is the pawns who put them in power.

"Be a queen of your own kingdom and never be a doormat- your voice is your own so use it and do not lose it"

"Popularity is not the most important thing in the world"

www.ingramcontent.com/pod-product-compliance
Lightning Source LLC
Chambersburg PA
CBHW051249020426
42333CB00025B/3120